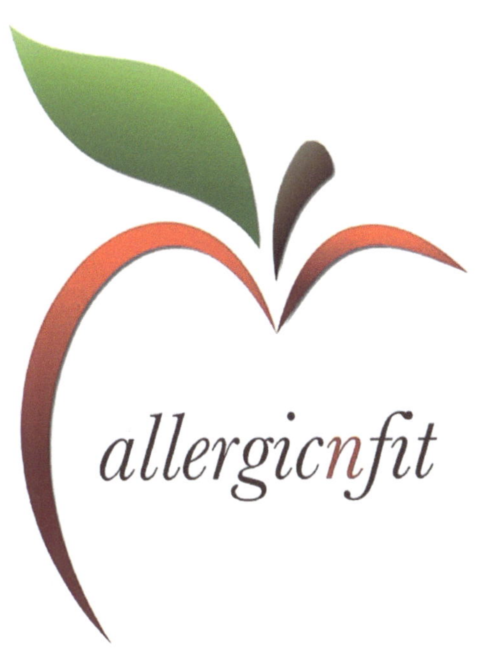


"Let food be thy medicine and medicine be thy food."
**Hippocrates**

I would like to thank my mother whom introduced me to cooking and enjoying it while pouring love into it. To my sister for helping me see my own strength. To my awesome daughter showing me, we all can accomplish what we love as long as we are resilient.

Thanks to everyone in my journey who helped me with knowledge, support and understanding.

Thank you all.

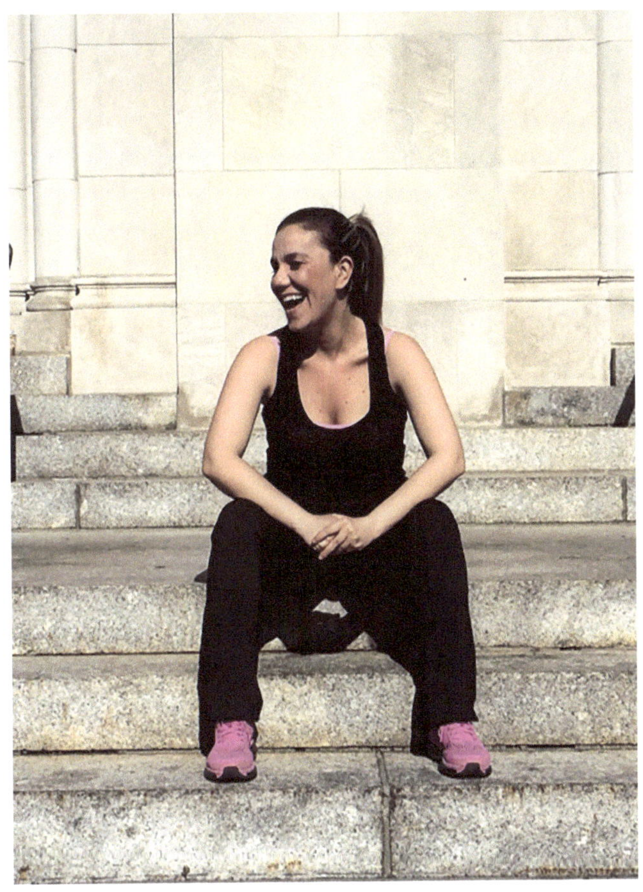

If you have only one smile in you give it to the people you love.

**Maya Angelou**

# PART 1

## *I NEED TO STOP EATING ALL THAT?*



This book is not intended as a substitute for the medical advice of physicians. The reader should consult a physician in all matters relating to his or her health.

I NEED TO STOP EATING ALL THAT?


Welcome to the new world of realization we are limited in our choices of food and yes, we need to stop eating our favorite slice of pizza or cake, but we can replace them with other options and even healthier ones.
At first it is hard, trust me I know, I really had a hard time as I entered this new world of cooking more often, reading labels, but being more conscious about what I ate made me feel better. Knowledge is power right!

How or why did I start eating gluten free? Well I was very sick and overweight I didn't feel good about myself at all. I know how it feels being at your job when it's lunchtime and you are scared to eat, because the selection of the food might not agree with you. There has been days I got really sick and ended up leaving work early, but I had no idea why the food I ate made me sick, or maybe there was another health reason. The symptoms were headache, nausea, diarrhea, gas, and bloating, total discomfort. I decided to go to the doctor, I had to find out why I kept feeling sick. I made an appointment and my journey started in year 2011.

As you know how it really goes when you are at a doctor's office, blood test, followed by urine test and if necessary more diagnostic tests. I have made appointments, followed my doctor's orders, went to all required tests, and the result was I was perfectly healthy. So here I am a healthy woman but I get sick whenever I eat. My episodes didn't stop and I never thought that the food I am eating was the reason. I kept feeling worse each day that passed by, and finally one day it finally dawned on me, it is the food I am eating that's making me sick. Now you have this confusing conversation in your head, 'how could all this be bad for me, I have been eating all these yummy stuff forever.'

Our body is a great machine; it gives us the signals and red lights if we really are in tune with ourselves. I was at a point in my life that whatever I ate made me sick, I mean like everything. I stopped eating all that I used to eat, and just ate potatoes with white meat, and slowly introduced other foods like vegetables and fruits one at a time, I had enough of being sick. Gluten has different symptoms on different people, but mostly it affects our digestive system in a nasty way.

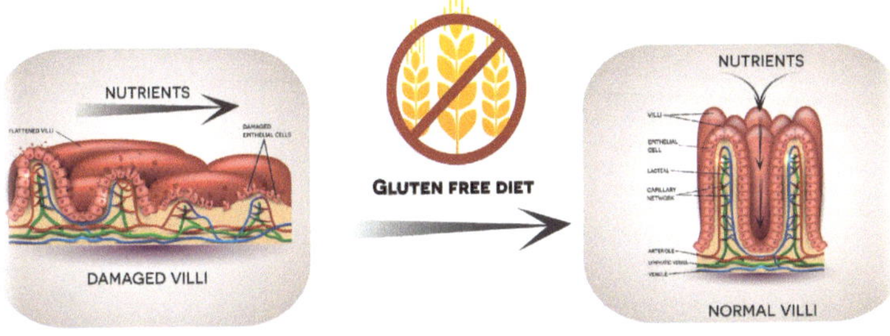



Millions of tiny finger-like structures
called villi, project inwards from the lining of
the small intestine. Damaged villi because of
Gluten consumption cause malnutrition and
digestive problems.

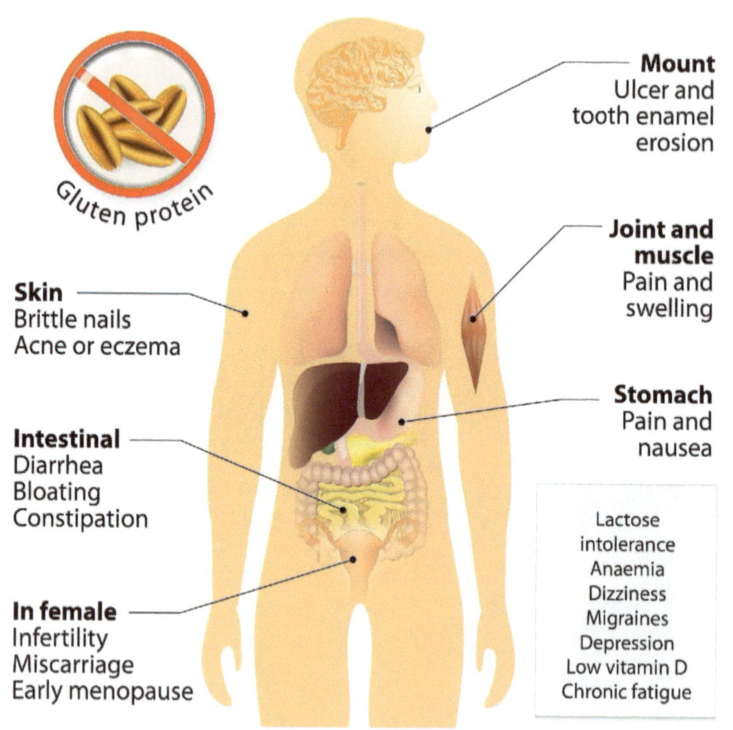


As I introduced different types of food one at a time I had different reactions and of course, all this takes time, like months, but I finally figured out what made me sick, GLUTEN. At that time, my immune system was so down, and my body was so out of order, my digestive system was really going crazy. Even though I finally figured out what was the real cause of my sickness, because of all that my body went through, I still couldn't eat certain things like eggs, red meat and cheese. I just couldn't digest them properly, and they also gave me discomfort. Here I am after the age of 30 years old, and now I have to change my diet, and what I eat completely. It was not easy, and yes, I did cheat on my diet because I just couldn't resist that muffin I had every morning for breakfast before work for years.

My body just kept reacting, I was in a battle with myself to change my eating habits, thought patterns, even the places I used to go and enjoy some delicious food.
 At that time as a person who had to eat gluten free, I didn't see many options, nor was there any gluten free products in the stores.
It was a struggle, but now when you look around you see gluten free products even in the stores in your neighborhood, like grocery stores and many people are getting more aware of food allergies, also the importance of healthy eating habits.

One thing I know it doesn't matter how easy it is to find products or restaurants to eat gluten free, if one does not change their habits of eating, it becomes even harder to change your life in a healthy way.
Here I am so proud of myself I figured out what my problem was, but now what? I am still overweight, and going through this new diet

regime I created for myself so I can be my healthy self again.

 I started my own research on dieting, as a person who never had any dieting experience in my life, it wasn't easy. I also started doing my research on supplementation about vitamins, fat loss products, and more importantly immune system boosters.


## What is Gluten?

Gluten is a storage protein found in wheat, barley and rye. Gluten can also be found in derivative of wheat, barley, and rye gains such as malt and brewer's yeast.

This was the start of my journey, and I was lucky to have a background on medical terminology, I am a certified Diagnostic Medical Sonographer, so in that sense, I was lucky in many ways. As I continued in my journey in exercise and supplementation I entered a different world I wasn't really familiar in. I decided to learn more and gather proper knowledge, so I enrolled to a personal training program from National Academy of Sports Medicine, and became a certified personal trainer. All the time, effort, and energy I have put in this journey has paid off, and now I can help others who are in my situation.

I can tell you from experience that talking to someone who can sympathize with you is good, but someone who is living through same issues as you do, is a shared experience, and exchange of knowledge with a pinch of emotion is the best.

Even though I was stuck with this limited diet and allergy for gluten, now I feel better than I did in my twenties. Why? Now I know more about how to be a healthy eater, and finally figured out those labels on the back of every food product there is. Back in the day I knew they were there, but never wondered why they were there, nor what they meant. Trust me, there are ingredients out there in our food that you wouldn't even want to get close to, let alone be consuming it.

My basic daily routine is I wake up, take my supplements before breakfast, have a light lunch, and have dinner preferably around 7pm, afterwards, I take my night time supplements before bed. I believe the combination of healthy, mental, emotional, and physical togetherness. Everybody has a different way of keeping their mental and emotional state healthy, I personally like short meditations, listening to music and workouts. Whatever works for you, we are all unique in our ways, what works for me maybe is not the right way for you. One thing I strongly recommend to everybody is walking, it is great to your body and your mind. Also, only consume natural/organic produce, I am not a fan of GMOs (genetically modified organisms) I like to eat what grows on earth, which is not enhanced or manipulated in any way.

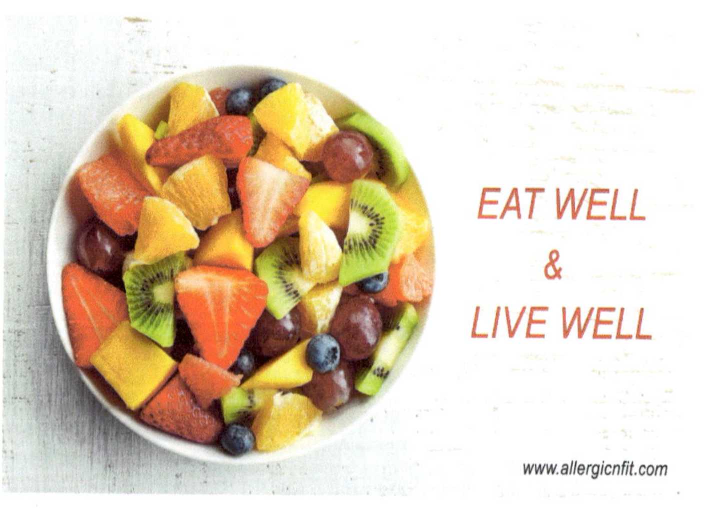

# Supplements

Supplements are a big part of my diet and during my healing process they were great help.

VITAMINS & SUPPLEMENTS

My Everyday Use

-Vitamin Code Women's Formula, Garden of Life (Men's for males)
- Once Daily Women's Probiotic, Garden of Life (Men's for males)

For Workouts
- Vega Sport Sugar-Free Energizer
- Isopure Zero Carb Protein Drink (ready to drink) or you can purchase the powder form.

There are many different companies producing different quality products, but these are what I use. You can always try different brands and find which is the right fit for you. I also strongly advise to consult your doctor before using any of these products, especially, if you have existing health conditions and using prescription medications.

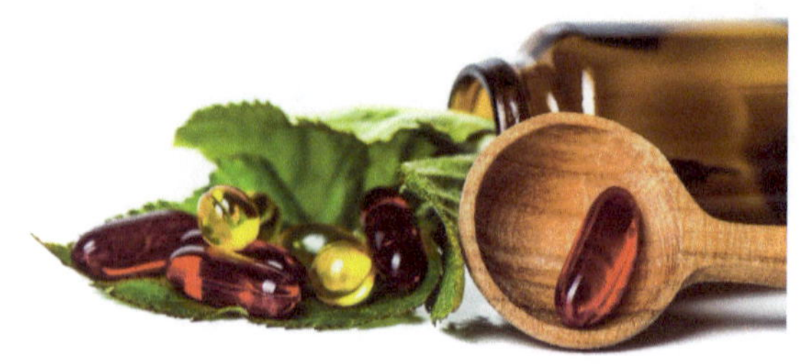

For weight loss, there are some products very useful and these are good to use as an aid to help you get to your desired weight, with good eating habits and some exercise of course. If we go back to the beginning our subject was, elimination of Gluten and allergy triggers for 4 to 8 weeks. Here are the helpful agents in healing the leaky gut, and all over healing digestive process.

You can purchase most of these products in health stores.


- Bone Broth
- Probiotics (boosting good bacteria in our gut will help our immune   system)
- Digestive Enzymes (aids in digestion, great remedy for food allergies)
 Enzymedica Digest Spectrum is a great product.
- L-glutamine (this an amino acid very effective repairing the gut and reducing intestinal inflammation)
   L-Glutamine Powder from Now Sports is a great product
- Coconut Oil  (for cooking, using in shakes and smoothies)
- Apple Cider Vinegar (2 tbsp in 8oz cup of water to drink or you can use on salads and meals)
 - We also want to lower our Candida in our gut the best product I have used is Solaray – Yeast Cleanse

## Avoid List

- Wheat starch
- Wheat bran
- Wheat germ
- Couscous
- Cracked wheat
- Durum
- Einkorn
- Emmer
- Farina
- Faro
- Graham flour
- Matzo
- Semolina
- Spelt
- Bulgur
- Oats (oats themselves don't contain gluten)
- Rye
- Barley

We need to read labels really carefully from salad dressings, to veggie burgers, seasonings, even all the way up to body lotions and makeup.

## Okay List

- Amaranth
- Arrowroot
- Buckwheat
- Cassava
- Millet
- Quinoa
- Rice
- Sorghum
- Soy
- Tapioca
- Corn
- Rice
- Fish
- Beef
- Chicken
- Seafood
- Fruits and vegetables
- Legumes
- Seeds
- Dairy products

Lets not forget our meat selection, grass fed and no antibiotics. For the rest of our food selection should be natural or organic.

I personally love and recommend almond or coconut milk, but it is okay to drink regular organic milk.

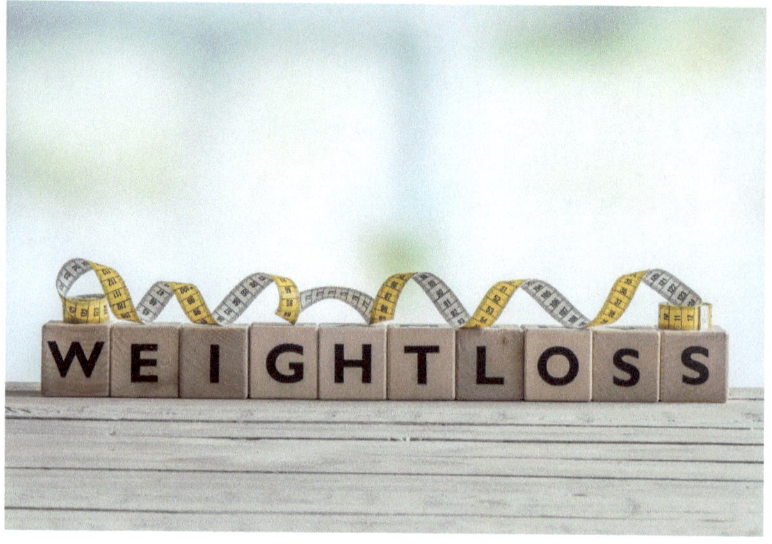


There are many different diets and ways to lose weight but in this chapter, I will be explaining about the ways I found useful in my own journey.

- Low Glycemic Diet

The glycemic index (GI) is a ranking system that classifies carb-containing foods by their effect on blood sugar levels. Dr. David Jenkins created it in the early 1980s.

- Intermittent Fasting

Intermittent fasting (IF) is an umbrella term for various diets that cycle between a period of fasting and non-fasting during a defined period. Intermittent fasting can also be used with calorie restriction for weight loss.

- The Ketogenic Diet

The Ketogenic Diet is simply consuming high-fat, good amount of protein and low carbs. No processed foods, high-carb foods and sugar.

# Low Glycemic Diet

## LOW GLYCEMIC
## 0-54 IDEAL

Apples          38
Apple juice          40
Apricots, dried 31
Bananas          54
Blueberries          25
Cherries          22
Coconut          45
Cranberries          45
Cranberry juice 50
Figs, dried          40
Grapefruit 25
Grapes          46
Orange juice          53
Oranges          44
Peaches          42
Pears, fresh          53
Plantains, raw 45
Plums          55
Strawberries          41

**Vegetables**

Artichokes 20
Asparagus 15
Bamboo shoots, raw 20
Beet greens 20
Broccoli 15
Broccoli rabe 10
Brussel sprouts 15
Butternut squash, baked 50
Cabbage, Chinese 10
Cabbage, savoy, boiled 15
Carrot juice 45
Carrots, raw 47
Cauliflower 15
Celery 15
Collard greens 20
Corn, sweet 54
Cucumber 15
Eggplant 15
Garlic 30
Green beans 15
Hubbard squash, baked 50
Kale 15
Leeks 15
Lettuce 15
Lima beans, baby, frozen 46
Okra, raw 15
Olives 15
Onions 15

Peppers 15
Pickles, dill 15
Turnip greens, boiled 10
Turnips, boiled 30
Snow peas 15
Summer squash 15
Tomato soup 54
Tomatoes  15
Spinach     15
Summer squash 15
Tomato soup 54
Tomatoes  15
Watercress        10
Zucchini     15

## Grains, Breads & Cereals
Gluten-free pasta 54
Basmati rice        50
Brown rice          50
Chickpeas  33
Quinoa       53
Gluten-free rice pasta 51

## Dairy and Dairy Alternatives
Skim milk 32
Soymilk 43
Yogurt, plain 14

**Nuts and Legumes**
Almonds   15
Black Beans         30
Broad beans         40
Butter beans         43
Cashews   23
Chickpeas  33
Fava beans          40
Horse beans         40
Kidney beans 41
Navy beans          54
Peanuts      14
Pinto bean 39
Soybeans, boiled 16
Split peas, yellow, boiled 45




Apricots, canned with light syrup 64
Apricots, fresh 57
Cantaloupe          65
Fruit cocktail 55
Grapes       66
Mango juice, unsweetened 55
Mangoes   56
Oranges      63
Orange juice 55

Papaya, fresh 55
Peaches, fresh 60
Peaches, canned 67
Pineapple   59
Raisins        64

## Vegetables
Marrowfat peas, dried 56
Peas, green        68
Sweet potato 61

## Grains, Breads & Cereals
Oat bran bread 68
Oatmeal, plain 58
Wild rice   57
Gluten-free corn pasta 68

## Dairy and Dairy Alternatives
Mayonnaise        60

## Nuts and Legumes
Black-eyed peas 59
Chestnuts 60
Lentil soup, canned    63
Pinto beans, canned 64

| | |
|---|---|
| Coca-Cola | 63 |
| Ketchup | 55 |
| Mustard | 55 |
| Nutella | 55 |
| Sushi | 55 |

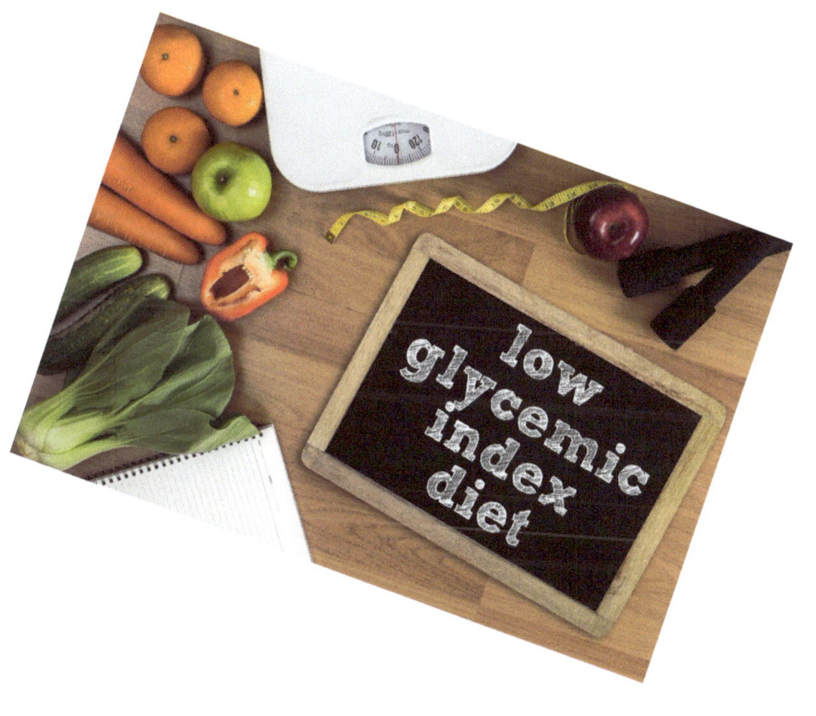

Dates   103
  Kiwifruit 75
  Watermelon 72

## Vegetables

Parsnips      139
Pumpkin      107
Rutabaga      103
Potato, instant      121
Potato, mashed      100
Potato, white, baked      85

## Grains, Breads & Cereals

Bagel      72
Bread stuffing 106
Gluten-free bread 90
Oatmeal      87
Rice cakes   82
Rice, brown 79
Rice, white  83
Tapioca, boiled with milk 115
Waffles      109
Gluten-free multigrain bread 79

## Dairy and Dairy Alternatives

Ice cream, full-fat  87
Ice cream, low-fat 71
Tofu, frozen dessert, non-dairy 164

Black bean soup 92
Green pea soup, canned 94
Kidney beans, canned 74
Lentils, canned 74
Split pea soup        86

**Snacks & Sweets**

Corn chips   105
Corn syrup   90
French fries 75
Jelly beans   80
Life Savers   70
Oatmeal cookies 79
Pastry        84
Popcorn 72


The healthiest weight loss is gradual, fast paced weight loss diets will help you lose weight, but afterwards hard to keep your desired weight.

The information above is an example of glycemic values of some delicious food. The main focus in this diet is to eat healthy, as you pick the right carbs to eat with your balanced diet.

When eating any type of carbohydrate our digestive system breaks it down into simple sugars that enter the bloodstream, all carbohydrates cause release of the hormone, insulin. This diet will help you choose the carbs wisely, and this way stabilize insulin levels.

By exchanging high-GI foods for low-GI alternatives, helps reducing blood sugar levels and promoting weight loss. This diet is a great healthy way, to lose weight and maintain weight loss.

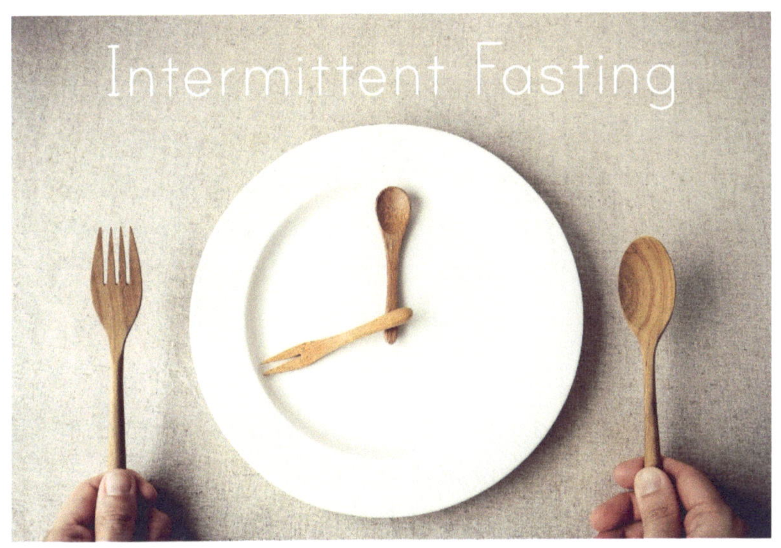


## Intermittent Fasting

There are different types of fasting.
Typical intermittent fasting times are generally from 14 to 18 hours. Even though some can fast anywhere from 32-36 hours, I would recommend 14 to 18 hours.

So what is intermittent fasting? In a very simple explanation, no food allowed during the times of fasting but you can enjoy water, coffee with no sugar or milk, and plain tea.

Let's say you are planning to fast 14 hours, you can start your fasting period right after dinner the night before. For example, dinner was at 7pm so no food before 12pm, lunchtime the next day. This way of fasting is easier because you are sleeping most of the time at night.

Also, after dinner you can workout, which is great for burning extra calories. At the beginning, you can start slowly by selecting 2 or 3 days of the week like Monday, Wednesday and Friday as fasting days.

One important factor is watching our calorie intake. Just because we fasted 14 hours, doesn't mean you can eat anything you desire afterwards. The best way is to eat healthy and nutritious food (ex: grilled chicken salad with a glass of iced tea, or if you prefer something lighter to break your fast, and you are unable to eat a meal, a protein shake is a good option.)

I can't stress enough, if you have a health condition please talk to your doctor before you start any diet or exercise regimen.

# KETO DIET
## FOOD PYRAMID

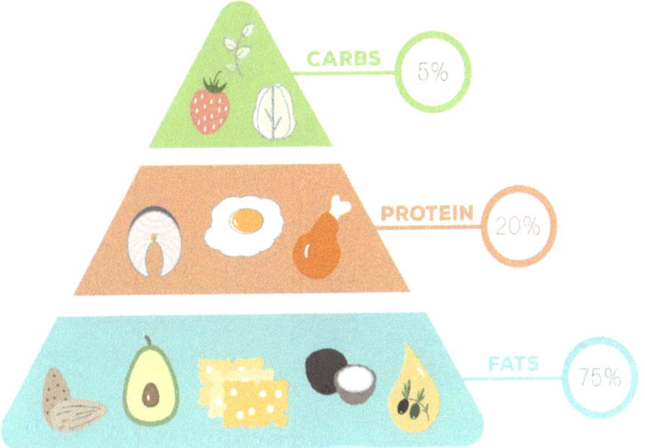


## The Ketogenic Diet

The Ketogenic diet is great for weight loss, especially when we need to stay away from gluten. Since the diet is low-carb, and the carbs that are consumed are vegetable based like leafy greens, makes life so much easier. The main focus in this type of diet, is making your body to become a fat burner instead of sugar burner.

In the process of being on this diet we go into the state of Ketosis. (Ketosis is a metabolic process, and it involves the body burning stored fat instead of glucose.) When we eat carbs, which results in production of glucose and insulin, which our bodies use for energy, the fats we consume are not used, nor needed causing fat storage. The Ketogenic Diet, eating low carbs, and changing the body's target for source of energy to fats, (which includes stored fats too) helps you get lean and healthy. What do we eat in this diet? Some examples are below.

## Healthy Fats

- Olive oil
- Coconut oil
- Flaxseed
- Avocados
- Butter
- Macadamia

## Proteins

- Beef, lamb, veal, liver etc. (grass-fed)
- Turkey, chicken, eggs, etc. (grass-fed)
- Salmon, tuna, sardines etc.  (wild caught)

## Vegetables

- Spinach, arugula, kale etc.
- Brussels sprouts, broccoli, cabbage etc.
- Celery, cucumber, zucchini, asparagus, green beans, bell peppers, tomatoes etc.

## Foods to Avoid

- Sugar, honey, agave, maple
- Corn, rice, cereal
- Potato, yams

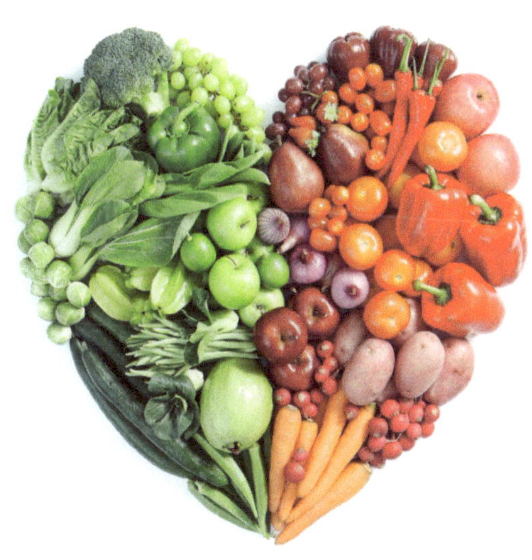

As you know there are many more options and ways of dieting and losing weight, the options I present are the ones I tried, and I think they are easier for anyone to do, especially those with gluten sensitivity, or allergy, who wants to get healthy and fit.

So you took a step and started eating healthy and completely eliminated gluten from your diet. You started a specific diet for weight loss and accomplished your goal for your desired weight, so now what? How do we keep the weight off and stay healthy? That's always been the dilemma, how do we keep our desired weight?

I believe diets work and the real difficulty comes after, when you stop dieting for weight loss. That's why dieting is a good stepping stone to lose weight, afterwards you always need to keep your healthy eating habits, which will become a way of healthy living.

Just keep your choices of food natural/organic, be aware of your portion sizes and stay away from sugar as best as you can, sugar really doesn't serve our body any good.

Always try to remember to read food labels, make your choices more on clean eating (no processed food) fruits, vegetables, and your choice of protein (fish, chicken, beef). Vitamins are a very important part of your health journey. Try to keep your meals balanced with healthy fats, protein and fiber, as much as nutritious food as you can. When you think you failed that day with your choices of food, just don't give up you can start over the next day. It's never been easy to change habits but motivation and consistency is the key. With effort and time you can make new habits to live a healthier life. We are what we repeatedly do, take initiative first, motivate yourself, reward yourself and keep going never give up. Once you form your new habits the rest is easy it comes natural without thinking about it, like buying your favorite cup of coffee every morning before work. We don't think about it. It's a habit developed over time and we just do it. The most important part is to believe in yourself, you can do anything you put your mind into. Trust me, I started from the beginning of changing everything and at first it wasn't easy, but new habits developed in time. Just like learning to walk, you fall and get up again and again, until you know how to walk.

# R E C I P E S

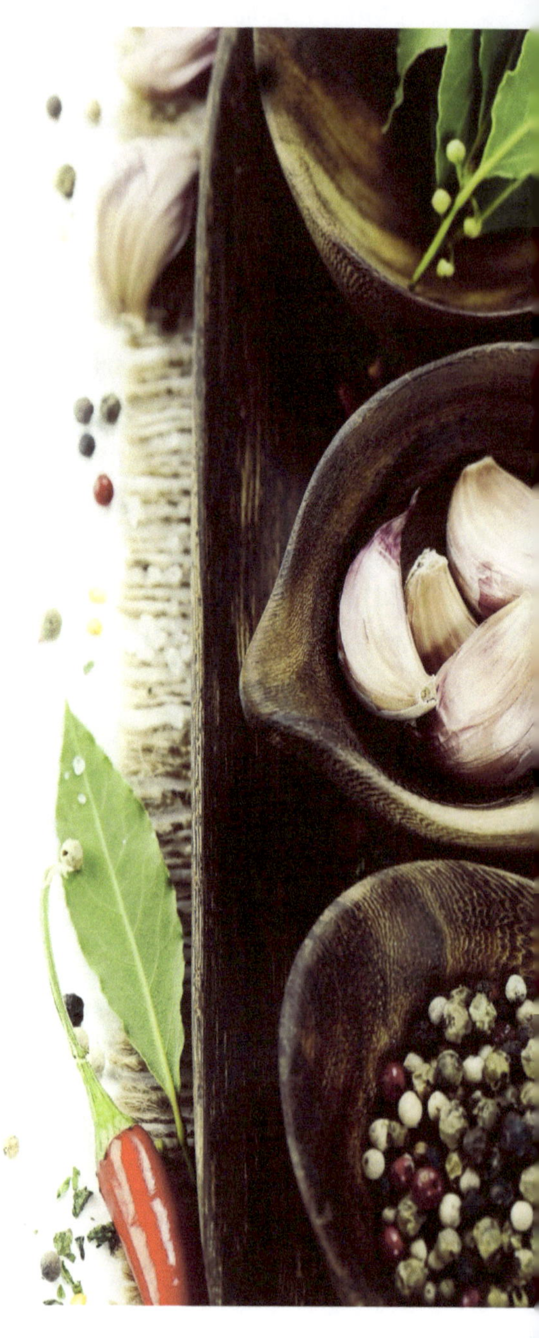

# Cucumber and Yogurt Dip

## Ingredients

- 2 cups of regular yogurt
- 1 cup cold water
- 1 tablespoon lemon juice
- 2 clove mashed garlic
- 4 (Persian) cucumbers, finely diced
- Pinch of salt
- 2 small bunches dried mint or fresh dill
- 1 tablespoon olive oil, to drizzle over the dip

## Instructions

1- First step, in a large bowl whisk yogurt, water and lemon juice.

2- Second step, we add mashed garlic, cucumbers, salt and dried mint or dill.

3- Now give it a good stir until all ingredients are mixed well. Drizzle oil on top.

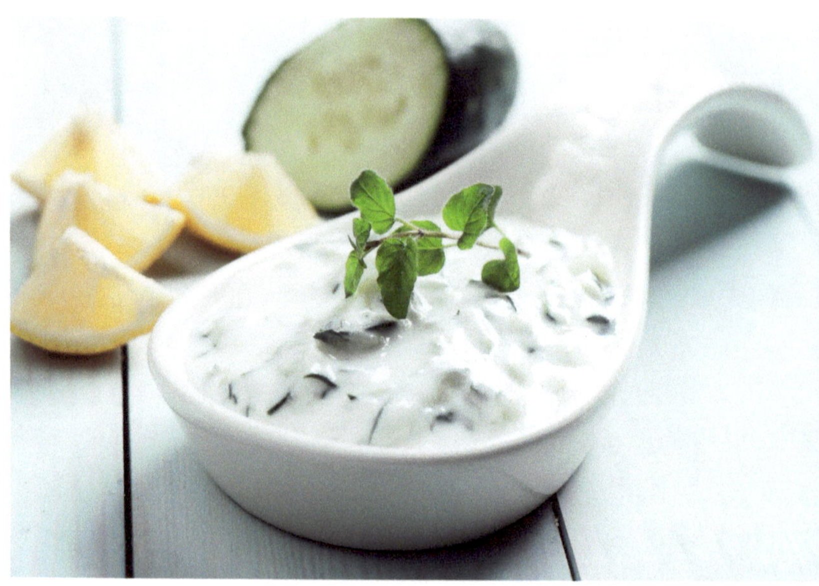

Tip: You can decorate with pieces of dill or fresh mint on top. I prefer putting minced dill in the mix instead of using dried mint. See which one is your favorite.

**Serving Size:** 4    **Prep time: 5 minutes**

# Scrambled eggs with peppers, onions and tomatoes

## Ingredients

- 2 tomatoes (medium size ripe, peeled and diced)
- 2 green Italian pepper (diced)
- 1 small onion (finely diced)
- 4 eggs lightly beaten
- 1 tbsp. butter
- Pinch of salt and black pepper
- Fresh mint or fresh dill if you want to decorate

## Instructions

1- First step, in a medium non-stick pan we put butter, onion and peppers. Season with salt and black pepper. Frequently stirring until ingredients are soft and changed color. Low heat is good throughout the cooking process

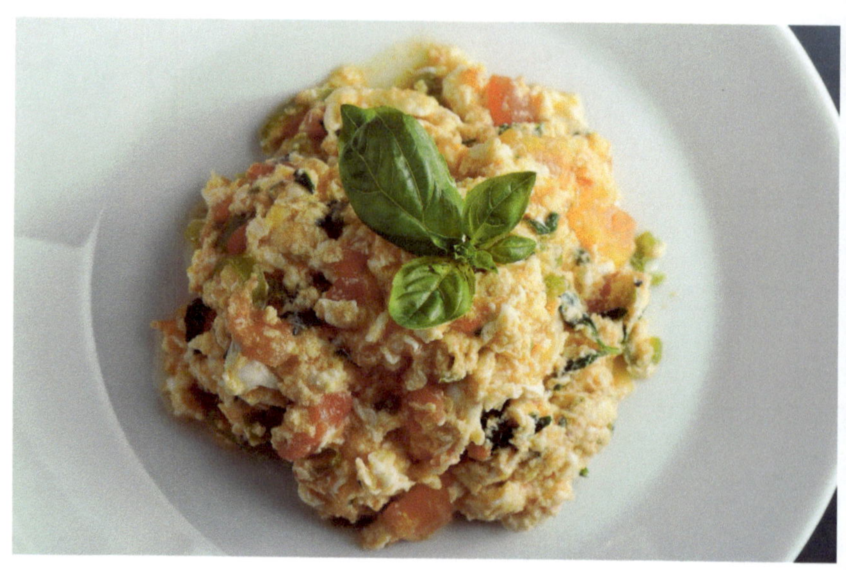

2- Second step we add the tomatoes and keep stirring until the tomatoes are cooked.


3-Third step is we add the lightly beaten eggs. It is best at this point to cover the pan until eggs are cooked.


**Serving Size:** 4

**Prep time: 15 minutes**

Red cabbage salad

## Ingredients

- 1/2 medium head red cabbage
- 1/2 cup olive oil
- 1 fresh lemon juice squeezed (or juice of half a lemon as you desire)
- 1 tbsp. salt
- 2 tbsp. apple cider vinegar

## Instructions

1- First step, chop the cabbage into small pieces.

2- Second step, we place the cabbage in a large bowl adding salt, lemon and vinegar.

3- Third step mix all the ingredients well.

**Serving Size: 6**     **Prep time: 15 minutes**

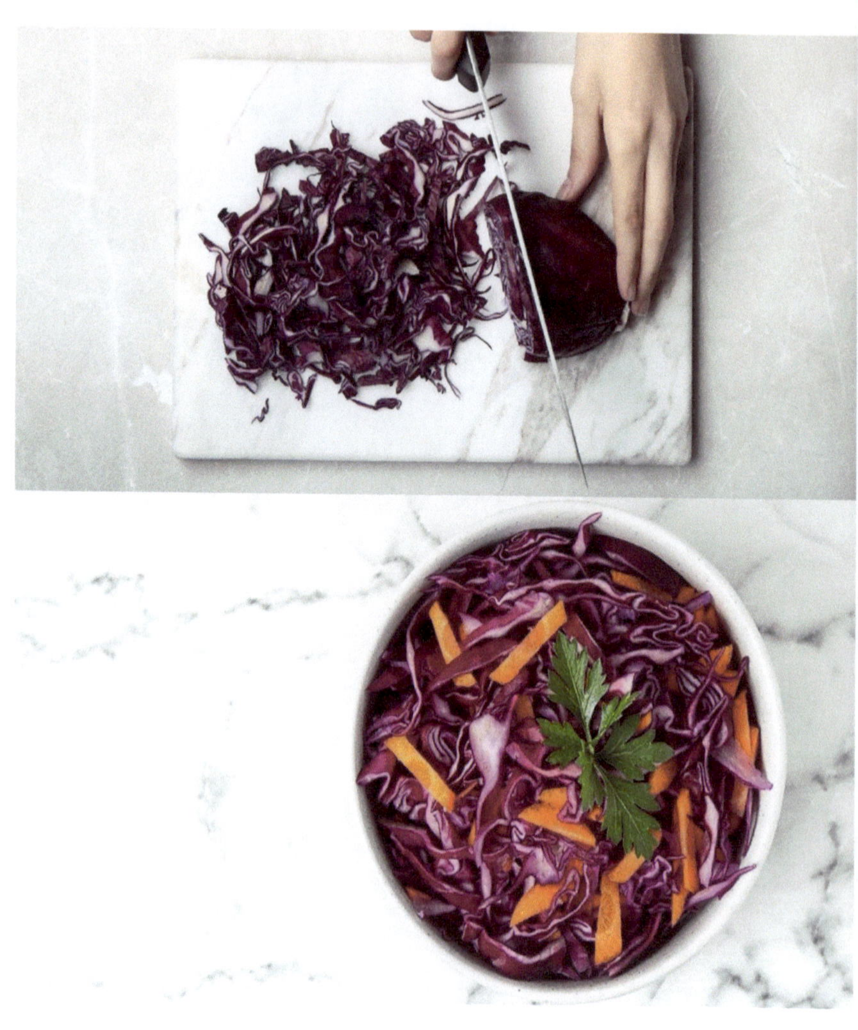

Tip: After adding lemon and oil if you wait a few minutes before serving, cabbage will be softer. Also you can add shredded carrots if you like a rich taste and add parsley on top.

## Ingredients

- 4 leeks chopped
- 2 carrots chopped
- 1 red onion diced
- 2 clove mashed garlic
- 5 tbsp. olive oil
- Pinch of salt
- 1 tbsp. white rice
- 1 tbsp. tomato sauce
- 1.5 cup water

## Instructions

1- First step, in a large pot we put olive oil and add onions stir them for a minute, than we add the tomato sauce and carrots, stir all for about 2 minutes.

2- Second step, we add the chopped leeks and salt in our pot, mix it all again.

3- Third step, add rice and water. You can turn off the stove after 20 minutes.

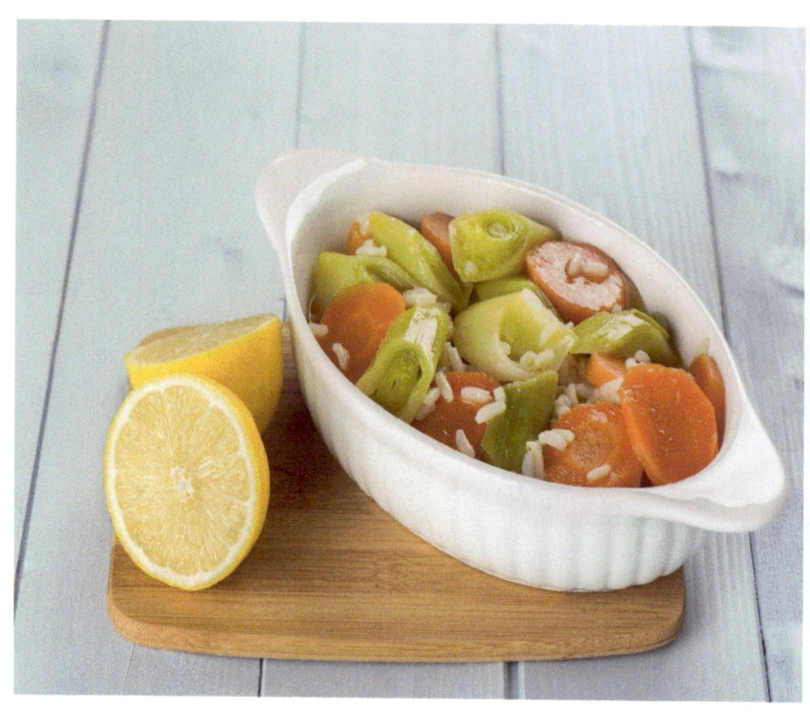

Tip: Serving warm or cold. Tastes great with some lemon.

**Serving Size:** 2          **Prep time:** 30 minutes

Pinto bean salad

## Ingredients

- 1 cup pinto beans (canned beans washed and drained)
- 4 leaves of romaine lettuce (chopped)
- 1 cucumber diced
- 2 small or medium size red pepper (chopped)
- 5 tbsp. olive oil
- Pinch of salt
- 1 fresh lemon juice squeezed (or juice of half a lemon as you desire)
- 1 handful fresh parsley and dill (chopped)
- 1 teaspoon dried mint

## Instructions

1- First step, in a large bowl we put beans, lettuce, red pepper, cucumber, parsley and dill.

2- Second step, we add the olive oil, lemon juice, salt and dried mint.

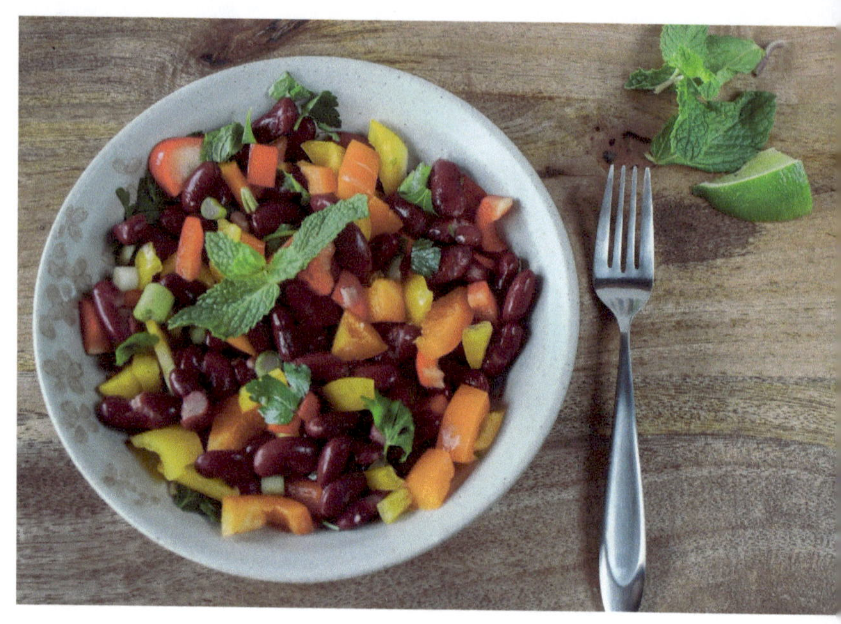

3- Third step, mix all the ingredients in the bowl well before serving.

Tip: For a colorful rich taste, you can add some colorful chopped bell peppers, cheese and/or olives.

**Serving Size:** 2          **Prep time:  15 minutes**

<h1 style="text-align:center">Potato salad with eggs</h1>

## Ingredients

- 4 medium size potatoes (boiled, peeled, chopped into cubes)
- 3 – 4 scallions, thinly sliced
- 2 boiled and peeled eggs
- 5 tbsp. olive oil
- 1 teaspoon salt
- 1/2 teaspoon black pepper
- 1 fresh lemon juice squeezed (or juice of half a lemon as you desire)
- 1 handful fresh parsley (chopped)

## Instructions

1- First step, in a large bowl we put our potatoes, olive oil, salt, pepper and mix them well.

2- Second step, we add parsley, scallions and lemon juice.

3- Third step is mixing all the ingredients in the bowl well. You may add eggs to the mixture.

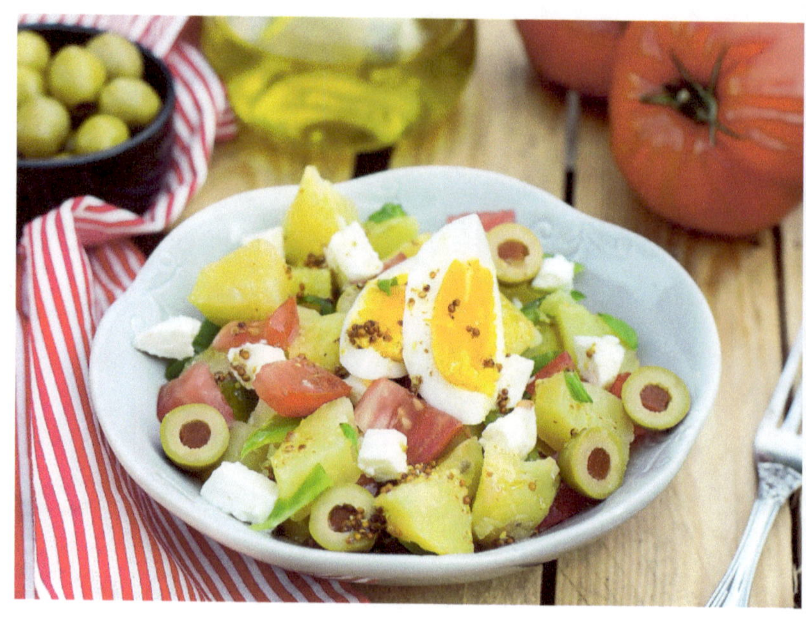

Tip: You can add some sliced pickles colorful chopped bell peppers, cheese and/or olives.

**Serving Size:** 4-6          **Prep time:**  20 minutes

## Ingredients

- 4 eggs (mixed in a bowl)
- 1 small red onion (chopped)
- 1 tbsp. olive oil
- ½ tbsp. butter
- 1/2 teaspoon salt
- 1/2 teaspoon black pepper
- 1/2 pack of white button mushroom (chopped)
- 1 handful fresh parsley (chopped)

## Instructions

1- First step, in a nonstick pan we put our olive oil, butter, chopped onions, salt, and black pepper. Stir it on medium heat until onions have a pinkish color.

2- Second step, we add the mushrooms to the pan and cook until mushrooms change color and are soft.

3- Third step, add the eggs to the mixture of mushrooms and onions in the pan.

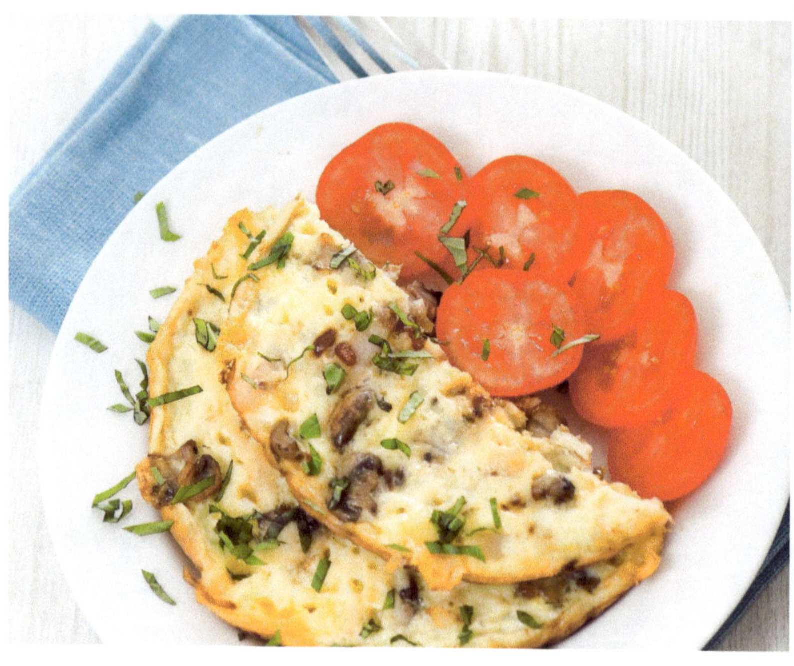

Tip: You can add some sliced tomatoes cheese and/or olives on the side before serving

**Serving Size:** 2-4          **Prep time:  10 minutes**

# Enjoy your life!

I hope you will enjoy the recipes I put some of my favorites, they are easy to cook, taste delicious and are diet friendly. You can always make your adjustment in ingredients (oil, salt, lemon etc) Cooking is great, if you are eating out most of the time I really advise you to start cooking at home. Start with easy recipes and the next thing you know you are a great cook.

Taking your supplements, watching your food intake, starting to cook at home, and exercising, are the main factors to accomplish your new healthy lifestyle.  For your fitness regime, walking is a great start you should do it everyday. In addition, I highly recommend light weight lifting. It doesn't matter which age group you fall under, light weight lifting keeps your muscles and bones strong. If you can go to the gym that's great, and if you can't whichever exercise routine you pick, do it gradually and consistently.
Do not stress yourself to be on a strict diet and a strict fitness program, just take one step at a time. I can tell you from experience we are more of what we eat, than how hard we workout, unless you want to be a bodybuilder.

---

There are other factors that affect our weight
like stress, lack of sleep, medications and
hidden health problems, are a few examples.
Do your best, be patient, if you fail today start
fresh tomorrow. Drink plenty of water and
please, use filtered water.

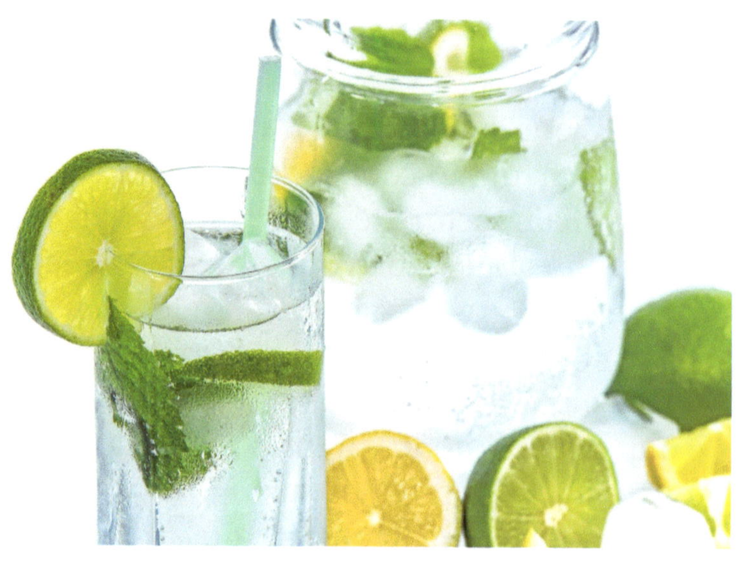

Water is our life source and it is very important
to stay hydrated for overall health. Stepping
into the new healthy lifestyle is a big and great
change, to be honest sometimes you can feel
stressed out during the process. At the end of
the road you are going to be so pleased with
your figure, your overall health, and you are
going to be so proud of yourself.

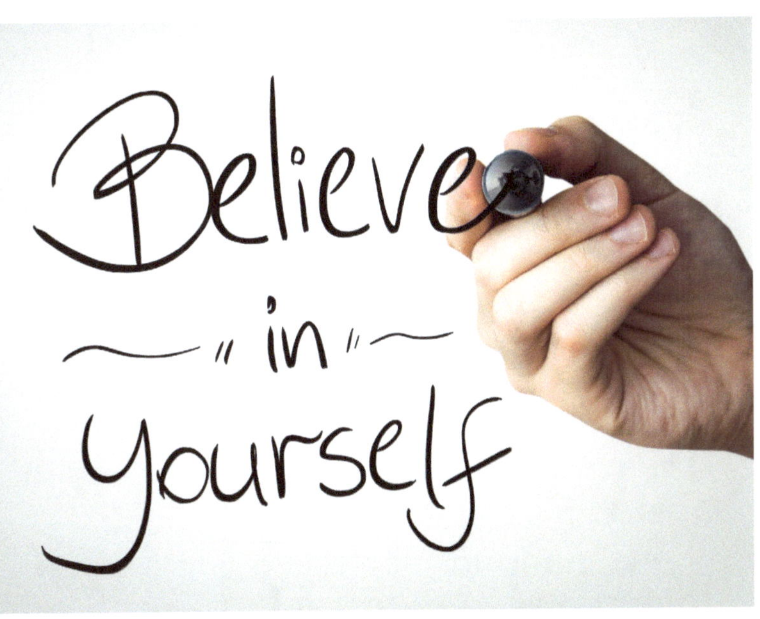


Everything takes time and patience, do not fall for the gimmicks in the market, people making false promises of rapid change (weight loss, muscle gain etc.) but we all know that great and stable changes take time. Your emotional health is also very important, as you know stress affects the human body very negatively, so it is important that you find outlets or hobbies that makes you happy, and most importantly enjoy your life to the fullest.

# LIST OF GLUTEN FREE PRODUCTS

These are a few examples of my favorites

- Schar
- Enjoy Life
- Glutino
- Ener-G Foods
- Udi's Gluten Free
- Goodpop
- Bragg Apple Cider Vinegar
- So Delicious Coconut Milk
- Van's Foods
- Kind Snacks
- Beetology
- Bakery on Main
- Bob's Red Mill
- Mary's Gone Crackers
- Nature's Path
- Larabar
- Rudi's
- Lundenberg Fmily Farms
- Applegate Farms
- Tate's Bake Shop

- Canyon Bakehouse
- Pure Organic
- Simole Mills
- Naturally Nutty
- Bfree Foods
- Khazana
- Namaste Foods
- Think Thin
- Aleia's
- Jane Bakes
- Deep River
- Ithaca Hummus
- Eden Organic
- Ian's

www.ingramcontent.com/pod-product-compliance
Lightning Source LLC
Chambersburg PA
CBHW041803260726
48664CB00034B/130